I0790928

TABLE OF CONTENT

Conclusion

CHAPTER ONE

It's time to take control
of your life!

Have you ever noticed
how we refer to babies
as 'the miracle of life',
yet often accept
mediocrity in our own
lives? What happened
along the way that made
us forget that we are
living a miracle? We
were told we could do
anything when we grew
up - so have you been
doing and having and

being everything you ever wanted?

Statistics show that the average American is 20 pounds overweight, in debt, depressed, and dislikes their job. Over time, many people settle for less than they truly want or deserve. However, there's no reason why you have to stay stuck in mediocrity. You can create the extraordinary life that everyone deserves- happiness, health, money, freedom, success and love.

It is possible to live your best life - your Level 10 life! It starts with how you wake up each morning and taking small steps every day to become the person you need to be for your desires. This book will help build three important arguments: (1) You are just as worthy and capable of creating success as anyone else on earth; (2) You must dedicate time each day to becoming better; (3) How you wake up dramatically affects all areas of your life. Even if you think you're not a morning person - The Miracle Morning will change all that!

CHAPTER TWO

Desperate search for
answers led him to
create a morning routine
that changed everything

I've been incredibly
lucky to have hit what
some might call "rock
bottom" twice in my
short life. I believe that
it was these challenging
and testing experiences
that gave me the ability
to create the life I
always dreamed of. And
I am forever grateful
that I can use not only
my triumphs but also
my failures to empower
and help others reach
beyond their boundaries
and achieve more than
they ever thought
possible.
My First Rock Bottom:
Dead at the Scene.

You may know, that my first rock bottom came when at 20 years old, I was hit head on by a drunk driver and died at the scene of the accident. This event, as well as the 8 life-changing lessons I learned from it, are detailed in my book, Taking Life Head On: How To Love the Life You Have While You Create the Life of Your Dreams.

My Second Rock Bottom: Deep In Debt and Deeply Depressed

My second plunge into despair was more taxing than dying in a car crash could have been. It was 2008, with the U.S economy suffering its worst recession since The Great Depression of the 30's. Despite building a great sales career, establishing a success coaching business with 6-figure profits, and writing a best-selling book - needless to say - money was an issue for me. My income had suddenly dropped in half and so debt piled up quickly. We were getting ready for our first child too, so all this led to deep emotional depression which eventually manifested into physical issues as well.

As unfortunate as it may sound, what got me through each day was knowing that at least I could crawl into bed in peace and momentarily escape from all my problems - thoughts of suicide circled around me regularly as well during this time... But deep down I knew that no matter how bad things were there would always be a way out of it. The Morning That Turned My Life Around. Then one morning - after taking advice from a friend - everything changed after going out on a run which I despised doing but did out of desperation; while listening to Jim Rohn's personal development audio something finally clicked within me when he said: "Your level of success will rarely exceed your level of personal development because success is so.

CHAPTER THREE

A 95% reality check:
why most people never
reach their fullest
potential, and what you
can do about it.

Every day we all face
the same challenge: to
reach our full potential
and not settle for
mediocrity. It's a
challenge to rise above
our excuses, do what's
right and create the
Level 10 life we want -
the one with no limits
that so few people ever
get to live. According to
the Social Security
Administration, if you
were to look at any 100
people at the start of
their working careers
and follow them for 40
years, you'd find that
only 1 will be wealthy,[4]

will be financially secure, 5 will continue working out of necessity, 36 will be dead and 54 will be broke and dependent on friends/family/governm ent. That means only 5% of us will live a life of true freedom while 95% will struggle their entire lives. So what can we do now to ensure we don't join this majority?

We must acknowledge that 95% of society never create or live the lives they really want - if we don't commit to thinking and living differently than most people then we too are doomed for a life of mediocrity. We can see this physically with obesity being an epidemic and

mentally/emotionally
with prescription drugs
being prescribed more
often than not in an
attempt to combat
disorders like
depression and anxiety.
Relationships suffer as
well with over half of
marriages ending in
divorce, while
financially Americans
are more in debt than
ever before while
spending more than they
should be earning.
The next step
understands why this
happens - why most
people end up
struggling - so that we
can prevent it from
happening to us. The
average person certainly
didn't plan on struggling
in life - so let's explore
what causes this
mediocrity!

CHAPTER FOUR

Why did YOU wake up this morning? Your mission, should you choose to accept it

Have you ever asked yourself why you get out of bed in the morning? Most people have to for one reason or another, but if given the choice, would we really want to? We hit the snooze button and resist waking up, unaware that our resistance might be sending signals that we'd rather stay in bed instead of creating the life we want. We may feel stuck and don't know how to break out of it.

The old proverb "You Snooze, You Lose" carries a deeper meaning than we may realize. When we delay getting out of bed until the last moment and hit the snooze button, we're actively resisting our life. Beginning your day with negative energy sets the tone for a cycle where feeling anxious or depressed tomorrow is more likely. People are missing out on a wealth of clarity and personal power that comes with waking up on purpose each morning. Those who do this join a small percentage of high achievers who are living their dreams.

Many experts will tell you there is no set amount of time as to how much sleep one needs; it varies between individuals and can be affected by genetics and health status. While some may need seven hours to feel their best, others may need nine hours. Contrary to popular belief, research has found that sleeping nine hours or longer is associated with negative outcomes such as illness or even death – this shows that too much sleep can be just as bad as not enough!

Rather than taking a scientific approach, I'm

going to focus on experiments from personal experience – what works for me might not work for you but give it a try anyway! I've found success in setting my intention to wake up every morning with enthusiasm for my day ahead. This has changed everything for me; I finally feel like I'm living my life rather than going through the motions and looking for escape from reality. You too can become the person you need to be in order to create the wealth, health, happiness, success, and freedom you desire if only you commit yourself!

CHAPTER FIVE

The 5-step snooze-proof wake up strategy (for the chronic snoozers)

I'm here to share a strategy that has helped me transform from sleeping through my alarm every morning, while believing I wasn't a "morning person", to now waking up early and feeling empowered to take on the day. Nobody really enjoys waking up early, but they do love the feeling they get after they have done it! To give yourself a motivation to wake up when your alarm clock goes off, I recommend following these five steps; they will make the process easier and help you significantly increase your Wake up Motivation Level (WUML).

Step #1: Set Your Intentions Before Bed - Your first thought in the morning is usually what you were thinking before you went to sleep, so it's important to create a positive expectation for the next morning. Download The Miracle Morning "Bedtime Affirmation" free at www.TMMBook.com for more help on this.

Step #2: Move Your Alarm Clock across the Room - Moving your alarm away from your bed helps force you out of bed and into motion;

motion creating energy will naturally help you wake up.

Step #3: Brush Your Teeth - Doing this simple activity will increase your WUML from a 1 or 2 to a 3 or 4.

Step #4: Drink a Full Glass of Water - After sleeping for 6-8 hours without water, dehydration can cause fatigue; drink water as fast as is comfortable for you and replace what was deprived from your body during sleep. This can take your WUML from 3 to 4 or 5.

Step #5: Get Dressed or Jump in the Shower - You can choose one of these two options; both of them will raise your WUML-5 or WULM-6, making it much easier to stay awake and do your Miracle Morning routine. Follow these five steps and you'll be able to drastically increase your Wake up Motivation Level!

CHAPTER SIX

These are a many unwelcome words that give a rather unfortunate, but fairly accurate description of how the average person feels about his or her life, far too frequently. You and I are really living in one of the most prosperous, advanced times in mortal history, with further openings and coffers available to us than ever ahead. Yet utmost of us are not tapping into the

unlimited eventuality
that's within every
single bone of us. I'm
not okay with that. Are
you? The Implicit Gap
Have you ever felt like
the life you want to live
and the person you
know you can be are
just beyond your grasp?
Do you ever feel like
you're chasing your
implicit you know it's
there, you can see it but
you can no way
relatively catch it?
When you see people
who are   outstripping in
an area that you 're not,
does it feel like they 've
got it all   figured out
like they must know
commodity that you do
not know, because if
you knew it, also you
'd be outstripping in
that area too? Utmost
of us live our lives on

the wrong side of a huge gap in our eventuality, a gap which separates who we are from who we can come. We're frequently frustrated with ourselves, our lack of harmonious provocation, trouble and results in one or further areas of life. We spend too important time allowing about the conduct we should be taking to produce the results that we want, but also we do not take those conduct. We all know what we need to do; we just do not constantly do what we know. Can you relate? This implicit gap varies in size from person to person. You may feel like you're veritably near your current eventuality and that a

many tweaks could
make all the difference.
Or you might feel the
contrary like your
eventuality is so far
down from who you 've
been that you do not
indeed know where to
start. Whatever the case
is for you, know that it's
absolutely possible and
attainable for you to live
your life on the right
side of your implicit
gap. Whether you're
presently sitting on the
wrong side of the grand
flume of your
eventuality, wondering
how you 're going to get
to the other side, or you
've been working your
way across the flume
but are stuck at a table
and have not been
suitable to close that gap
and get to the coming
position this chapter

will introduce you to six
tools that will enable
you to go from where
you are accepting lower
from yourself than what
you know is possible to
developing yourself into
the person you know
you can come. Your
Life Is Not What You
suppose It Is utmost of
us are so busy trying to
manage, maintain, or
indeed just survive our
life " situation " that we
do not make the time to
concentrate on what's
most important our life.
What's the difference?
Our life   situation is
the set of external
circumstances, events,
people, and places that
compass us. It's not
who we are. We're
further than our life
situation. Your life is
who you're at the

deepest position. Your life is made up of the internal factors, stations, and mindsets that can give you the power to alter, enhance, or change your life situation at any given moment. Your life is made up of the Physical, Intellectual, Emotional, and Spiritual corridor that make up every human being or P.I.E.S. for short. The Physical includes effects like your body, health, and energy. The Intellectual incorporates your mind, intelligence, and studies. The Emotional takes into account your feelings, passions, and stations. The Spiritual includes intangibles similar as your spirit, soul, and the unseen advanced power that oversees all. Your l i f e is where your capability to produce new passions, perspectives, beliefs, and stations in your " inner " world lies, so that you can produce or alter the circumstances, connections, results, and anything differently in the " external " realm of your life situation. As numerous pundits have tutored us our external world is a reflection of our inner world. In other words, by fastening time and trouble each day on developing your P.I.E.S., and constantly getting a better interpretation of yourself, your life situation will inescapably nearly automatically ameliorate. I can assure you that through my own transformative trip from the depths of mediocrity, justifying my defenses and living most areas of my life nearly in between medium and average, to achieving pretensions that at one time sounded insolvable for me your commitment to diurnal particular development will be as necessary for your metamorphosis as it was for mine.

For far too numerous people, they miss out on the extraordinary, full, rich life they really want- our 10th position life- because they get overwhelmed by the circumstances of everyday life. Her living situation took up so much of her time that her life, most importantly, was neglected. To help your 10th position life from being neglected and limited by the demands of your life situation- eventually leading to a life of remorse, unfulfilled eventuality, or indeed mediocrity- you must prioritize and invest time in particular growth every day. Enter The Miracle Morning Life SAVERS- a set of six simples, life-enhancing, life-changing diurnal practices, each of which develops one or further physical, intellectual, emotional, and spiritual aspects of your life so you can come You yourself need to produce the life you want.

Nope, it's not "sleep," Sorry. While I know numerous people would love it if they could sleep their way to success, unless you have been cryogenically firmed and are awaiting a large heritage at the time of being fused out life just does not work that way. There are six important, proven particular development practices known as the Life S.A.V.E.R.S. that you'll use to gain access to the important forces formerly within you that will enable you to alter, change, or transfigure any area of your life. Let's look at each of the six particular development tools that make up the Life S.A.V.E.R.S. and how each will help you come the person you need to be to fluently attract, produce, and live the most extraordinary life you have ever imagined.

Nope, it's not "sleep." Sorry. While I know multitudinous people would love it if they could sleep their way to success, unless you have been cryogenically concrete and are awaiting a large heritage at the time of being fused out life just does not work that way. Also are six important, proven particular development practices known as the Life S.A.V.E.R.S. that you'll use to gain access to the important forces formerly within you that will enable you to alter, change, or transform any area of your life? Let's look at each of the six particular development tools that make up the Life S.A.V.E.R.S. and how each will help you come the person you need to be to easily attract, produce, and live the most extraordinary life you have ever imagined. Do you invest time in centering yourself and creating an optimum state of mind to lead you through the rest of the day? Or do you generally stay to wake up until you've got commodity to do? Does the words calm, peaceful, or invigorating describe your average morning? If they do, congratulations! You're formerly a step ahead of the rest of us. For utmost of us, words like rushed, excited, stressful or indeed chaotic might best describe our typical morning. For others, laggardly, lazy, and sleepy might be a more accurate description of how the morning begins. Which of these scripts stylish describes your average morning? Mornings, for utmost of us, are generally enough excited and rushed. We 're generally running around trying to get ready for the day, and our minds are frequently agonized with internal chatter about what we've to do, where we've to go, who we've to see, what we forgot to do, the fact

that we 're running late,
a recent argument with
our significant other or
family member.

For others, we've
trouble just getting
going on utmost
mornings. We feel
sluggish, lazy, and
unproductive. So, for
the great maturity of us,
the mornings are
moreover stressful and
rushed, or slow and
unproductive. Neither of
these represents the
optimum way to start
your day. Silence is one
of the stylish ways to
incontinently reduce
stress, while adding
your tone- mindfulness
and gaining the clarity
that will allow you to
maintain your focus on
your pretensions,
precedence's, and

what's most important
for your life, each and
every day. There are
some of my favorite
conditioning to choose
from and practice
during my period of
Silence, in no particular
order, followed by a
simple contemplation to
get you started:
Meditation, Prayer,
Reflection, Deep
Breathing, and
Gratitude. Some
mornings I do just one
of these conditioning,
and other mornings I
combine them. All of
these practices will
relax your mind and
body, calm your spirit,
and allow you to be
completely present and
open to entering the
benefits that will come
from the remaining Life
S.A.V.E.R.S. which

make up the rest of your Miracle Morning. It's veritably important that you do not stay in bed for this, and   rather that you leave your bedroom altogether. The problem with staying in bed or indeed in your bedroom, where your comfy bed is within your line of sight is that it's too easy to go from sitting in Silence, to limping, to falling back asleep. I always sit on my living room settee, where I formerly have everything set up that I need for my phenomenon Morning. My declarations, journal, yoga DVD, the book I 'm   presently reading everything has its place and is ready for me each day so that, in the morning, it's easy to jump right in and engage in my phenomenon Morning, without having to search for anything. Contemplation Since there are plenitude of great books, papers, and websites that concentrate on contemplation, I won't go into too important detail in describing the proven benefits and the colorful approaches to planning. Rather, I'll just mention a many of what I believe are the most significant benefits, and give you simple step- by- step contemplation that you can begin incontinently. The substance of contemplation is simply silencing or fastening the mind for a period of time. You may or may not be apprehensive of all the extraordinary health benefits of planning. Study after study shows that contemplation can be more effective than drug. Studies link regular contemplation to changes in metabolism, blood pressure, brain activation, and other mind and fleshly functions. It can palliate stress and pain, promote sleep, enhance focus and attention, and indeed increase lifetime. Contemplation also requires veritably little time. You can take advantage of the benefits of contemplation in just a many twinkles a day. Well- known celebrities, CEOs and largely successful people like

Jerry Seinfeld, Sting, Russell Simmons, Oprah and numerous further have publically stated that regular, frequently daily, contemplation has come an inestimable part of their life. Tupperware CEO Rick Goings told The Financial Times that he tried to meditate for at least 20 twinkles every day, stating, "For me, it's a practice that not only burns off stress, but gives me fresh eyes to clarify what's really going on and what really matters." Oprah told Dr. Oz that Transcendental Meditations has helped her "connect with that which is God," according to the Huffington Post. There are numerous stripes and types of contemplation, but generally speaking you can divide them into two orders " guided " and " individual " contemplations. Guided contemplations are those in which you hear to another person's voice and admit instructions to help guide your studies, focus, and mindfulness. Individual contemplations are simply those you do on your own, without backing from anyone differently. Phenomenon Morning Contemplation. Then a simple, step- by- step individual contemplation that you can use during your Miracle Morning, indeed if you 've no way meditated ahead. Before beginning your contemplation, it's important to prepare your mindset and set your prospects. This is a time for you to quiet your mind and let go of the obsessive need to constantly be allowing about commodity either reliving the history, stressing or fussing about the future but no way living completely in the present. This is the time to let go of your stresses, take a break from fussing about your problems, and be completely present in this moment. It's a time to pierce the substance of who you truly are to go deeper than what you have, what you do, or the markers you 've accepted as " who you are " which utmost people have no way indeed   tried to do. Penetrating this substance of who you truly are is   frequently appertained to as "just being." Not allowing, not doing, and just being. However, or too "new- age" that's okay, If this sounds foreign to you. I used to feel the same way. It's presumably just because you've no way tried it ahead. But thankfully, you're about to. I'm the topmost! " Muhammad Ali affirmed these words over and over again and also he came them. Declarations are one of the most effective tools for snappily getting the person you need to be to

achieve everything you
want in your life.
Declarations allow you
to design and also
develop the mindset
(studies, beliefs, focus)
that you need to take
any area of your life to
the coming position. It's
no coexistence that
some of the most
successful people in our
society celebrities like
Will Smith, Jim Carrey,
Suez Orman,
Muhammad Ali, Oprah,
and numerous further
have each been oral
about their belief that
positive thinking and
the use of declarations
has helped them on their
trip to success and
wealth. Whether or not
you realize it, constantly
talking to one's tone is
not just for crazy
people. Every single one

of us has an internal dialogue that runs through our heads, nearly one-stop. Utmost of its unconscious, that is, we do not purposely choose the dialogue. Rather, we allow our once gests both good and bad to renewal over and over again. Not only is this fully normal, it is one of the most important processes for each of us to learn about and master. Yet, veritably many people take responsibility for laboriously choosing to suppose positive, visionary studies that will add value to their lives. I lately read a statistic that 80 of women have tone-disapproving studies about themselves (body image, job performance,

other people's opinion
of them, etc.)
throughout the day. I 'm
sure that men do also,
although it may be to a
lower extent. Your
tone- talk has dramatic
influence on your
position of success in
every aspect of your life
confidence, health,
happiness, wealth,
connections, etc. Your
declarations are
moreover working for
or against you,
depending on how
you're using them. If
you do not purposely
design and choose your
declarations you're
susceptible to repeating
and reliving the fears,
precariousness, and
limitations of your
history. still, when you
laboriously design and
write out your

declarations to be in alignment with what you want to negotiate and who you need to be to negotiate it and commit to repeating them   diurnal (immaculately out loud) they incontinently make an print on your subconscious mind. Your declarations go to work to transfigure the way you suppose and feel so you can overcome your limiting beliefs and actions and replace them with those you need to succeed. My first real- life exposure to the power of declarations came when I was living with one of my most successful musketeers, Matt Recore. Nearly every day, I would hear Matt crying from the shower in his bedroom. Allowing he was yelling for me, I would approach his bedroom door, only to find that he was crying effects like, "I'm in control of my fortune! I earn to be a success! I'm committed to doing everything I must do moment to reach my pretensions and produce the life of my dreams! " What a codger, I allowed. The only former exposure I had to declarations was through a popular 1990s imitate on the hit television show Saturday Night Live, in which Al Franken's character Stuart Smalley used to gawk into a glass and reprise to himself, " I 'm good enough, I 'm smart enough, and doggone it, people like me! " As a result, I always allowed of declarations as a joke. Matt knew better. As a pupil of Tony Robbins, Matt had been using declarations and conjurations for times to produce extraordinary situations of success. Retaining five homes, and one of the top network masterminds in the country (each by age 25), I should have figured Matt knew what he was doing. After all, I was the one renting a room in his house. Unfortunately, it took me a many further times to realize that declarations were one of the most important tools for transubstantiating your life. My first-hand experience using declarations came when I read about them in Napoleon Hill's fabulous book, suppose and Grow Rich(which I largely recommend, by the way). Although I was skeptical that the reiteration of declarations was really going to make any measurable impact on my life, I allowed i would give it a shot. However, it might work for me, if it worked for Matt. I chose to target the limiting belief I had developed after suffering significant brain damage in my auto accident I've a horrible memory. Still, Taking Life Head On! You know that if you read my firstbook.my short term memory was nearly missing following my auto accident. While this led to some suitable comical incidents, my memory was so poor that musketeers and family would spend hours visiting with me at the sanitarium, take a quick lunch break, and also return to have me hail them as if I had not seen them in times. Facing such a real physical limitation due to a traumatic brain injury caused me to constantly support the belief that I've a horrible memory. Anytime someone asked me to flash back or remind them of commodity, I would always respond, "I would, but I really cannot, I've brain damage and a horrible short- term memory."

It had been 7 times since my auto accident, and while this belief was grounded on my reality also, it was time to let it go. Perhaps my memory was so horrible, at least in part, because I had no way made the trouble to believe it could ameliorate. As Henry Ford said, "Whether you suppose you can, or you suppose you cannot, you're right either way. "Still, to me, the most justified if declarations could change what was. Limiting belief that I had, also they could presumably change anything. So, I created my first protestation which read I'm letting go of the limiting belief that I have a horrible memory. My brain is a

miraculous organism
able of healing itself,
and my memory can
ameliorate, but only in
proportion to how
important I believe it
can ameliorate. So,
from this moment on,
I'm maintaining the
unwavering belief that
I've an excellent
memory, and it's
continuing to get better
every day.   I read this
short protestation every
day, during my
phenomenon Morning.
Still programmed with
my once beliefs, I was
not sure it was working.
Also, two months after
my first day reciting my
protestation, commodity
passed that had not
passed in over seven
times. A friend asked
me to flash back to call
her the coming day, and

I responded, "Sure, no problem." As soon as the words left my mouth, my eyes widened and I got agitated! My limiting belief about my horrible memory was losing its power. I had replaced it and reprogrammed my subconscious mind with my new, empowering belief, using my declarations. From that point on, having also added the belief that declarations really work, not only did my memory continue to ameliorate, but I created declarations for every area of my life that I wanted to advance. I began using declarations to ameliorate my health, finances, connections, overall happiness, confidence, as well as

any and all beliefs,
mindsets and habits that
demanded an upgrade.
Nothing was off limits.
There are no limits!
We've each been
programmed at the sub-
conscious position to
suppose, believe, and
act the way we do. Our
programming is a result
of numerous influences,
including what we've
been told by others,
what we've told
ourselves, and all of our
life gests both good and
bad. Some of us have
programming that
makes it easy for us to
be happy and
successful, while others
conceivably the
maturity have
programming that
makes life delicate. So,
the bad news is that if
we do not laboriously

change our
programming, our
eventuality will be
crushed and our lives
limited by the fears,
precariousness, and
limitations of our
history. We must stop
programming ourselves
for a life of mediocrity
by fastening on what
we 're doing wrong,
being too hard on
ourselves when we
make miscalculations,
and causing ourselves to
feel shamefaced, shy,
and undeserving of the
success we really want.
The good news is that
our programming can be
changed or   bettered at
any time. We can
reprogram ourselves to
overcome all of our
fears, precariousness,
bad habits, and any
tone- limiting, implicit-

destroying beliefs and actions we presently have, so we can come as successful as we want to be, in any area of our lives we choose. You can use declarations to start programming yourself to be confident and successful in everything you do, simply by constantly telling yourself who you want to be, what you want to negotiate and how you're going to negotiate it. With enough reiteration, your sub-conscious mind will begin to believe what you tell it, act upon it, and ultimately manifest it in your reality. Putting your declarations in writing makes it possible for you to choose your new programming so it moves you towards that asked condition or state of mind by enabling you to constantly review it. Constant reiteration of a protestation will lead to acceptance by the mind, and affect in changes in your studies, beliefs and actions. Since you get to choose and produce your declarations, you can design them to help you establish the studies, beliefs, and actions that you want and need to succeed.

Five Simple Ways To Produce Your Own Declarations

There are five simple way to produce your first protestation, followed by a link where you can download free Miracle Morning declarations.

Step 1: What You Really Want The purpose of a written protestation is to program your mind with the beliefs, stations, and actions habits that are vital to your being suitable to attract, produce, and to sustain your ideal situations of success position 10 successes in every area of your life. So, your protestation must first easily eloquent exactly what you want your ideal life to be like, in each area. You can organize your declarations according to the areas that you most want to concentrate on perfecting, similar as

Health/ Fitness,
Mindset, feelings,
Finances, connections,
Church, etc. Begin with
clarifying, in jotting,
what you really want
your ideal vision for
yourself and your life in
each area.

Step 2: Why You Want
it as my good friend
Adam Stock, President
of Rising Stock, Inc.
formerly told me, "The
wise begin with whys."
Everyone wants to be
happy, healthy, and
successful, but wanting
is infrequently an
effective strategy for
getting. Those who
overcome the
temptations of
mediocrity and achieve
everything they want in
life have an
extraordinarily

compelling why that drives them. They've defined a clear life purpose that's more important than the collaborative sum of their petty problems and the innumerous obstacles they will inescapably face, and they wake up each day and work towards their purpose. Include why, at the deepest position, all of the affects you want are important to you. Being demitasse clear on your deepest whys will give you an impregnable purpose.

Step 3: Whom You Are Committed to being to produce It As my first Coach, Jeff Sooey used to say, this is where the rubber meets the road.
In other words, your life

gets better only after you get better. Your external world improves only after you've invested innumerous hours perfecting yourself. Being (who you need to be) and doing (what you need to do) are prerequisites for having what you want to have. Get clear on who you need to be, are committed to being, in order to take your life, business, health, marriage, etc. to the coming position and beyond.

Step 4: What you're Committed to Doing to Attain It Which conduct will you need to take on a harmonious base to make your vision for your ideal life a reality? Want to lose weight?

Your protestation might say commodity like I'm 100 married to going to the spa 5 days a week and running on the routine for a minimum of 20minutes.However, your protestation If you're a sales person. Might read I 'm committed to making 20 prospecting calls every day, from 8am-9 am. The more specific your conducts are the better. Be sure to include frequency (how frequently), volume(how numerous), and precise time frames(what times you 'll begin and end your conditioning.) It's also important to start small. If you're going to the spa 0 days a week for 0 twinkles, going to 5 days a week for 20 twinkles is a big vault. It's important to take manageable way. Feel small successes along the way so you feel good and do not get discouraged by setting prospects too high to be suitable to maintain. You can make up to your ideal thing. Start by writing down a diurnal or daily thing and decide when you will increase it. After a many weeks of successfully meeting your thing of going to the spa 2- days-a-week for 20 twinkles, also move it up to 3- days-a-week for 20 twinkles, and so on.

Step 5: Add Inspirational quotations and doctrines I'm always on the lookout for quotations and doctrines that I can add to my declarations. For illustration, one of my declarations comes from the book What Got You Then Won't Get You There by Marshal Goldsmith. It reads, "The# 1 skill of influencers is the sincere trouble to make a person feel that he or she's the most important person in the world. It's one of the chops that Bill Clinton, Oprah Winfrey, and Bruce Goodman used to come the stylish in their fields. I'll do this for every person I connect with! " Another reads " Follow Tim Ferris 'advice To maximize productivity, schedule 3- 5 hour blocks or half-days of singularly concentrated attention on ONE single exertion or design, rather than trying to switch tasks every 60 twinkles. ” Anytime you see or hear a quotation that inspires you, or come across an empowering gospel or strategy and suppose to yourself Man that is a huge area of enhancement for me, add it to your declarations. By fastening on these every day, you'll begin to integrate the empowering doctrines and strategies into your way of thinking and living, which will ameliorate your results and quality of   life.

In order for your declarations to be effective, it's important that you tap into your feelings while reading them. Mindlessly repeating a expression over and over again, without feeling its verity, will have a minimum impact on you. You must take responsibility for generating authentic feelings and forcefully investing those feelings into every protestation you repeat to yourself. Have fun with it. However, it does not hurt to If you're agitated about an protestation. Cotillion and roar it from the rooftops! It can also be salutary to incorporate a purposeful physiology,   similar as reciting your declarations while standing altitudinous, taking deep breaths,

making a fist, or
exercising. Combining
physical exertion with
declarations is a great
way to harness the
power of the mind-
body connection. Keep
in mind that your
declarations will no way
really be a "final" draft,
because you should
always be streamlining
them. As you continue
to learn, grow, and
evolve, so should your
declarations. When you
come up with a new
thing, dream, habit, or
gospel you want to
integrate into your life,
add it to your
declarations. When you
negotiate a thing or fully
integrate a new habit
into your life, you might
find it's no longer
necessary to
concentrate on it every

day, and therefore choose to remove it from your declarations. Eventually, you must be harmonious with reading your diurnal declarations. That's right, you must read them daily. Saying an occasional protestation is as effective as getting an occasional drill. You won't see any measurable results until you make them a part of your diurnal routine. That's largely what The Miracle Morning 30 Day Life Transformation Challenge (in Chapter 9) is all about making each of the Life S.A.V.E.R.S. a habit so you can   do them painlessly. One further thing to consider reading this book or any

book is a protestation
to you. Anything you
read influences your
studies. When you
constantly read positive
tone- enhancement
books and papers, you're
programming your mind
with the studies and
beliefs that will support
you in creating success.
Visualization, also
known as creative
visualization or internal
trial, refers to the
practice of seeking to
induce positive results
in your external world
by using your
imagination to produce
internal film land of
specific actions and
issues being in your life.
Constantly used by
athletes to enhance their
performance,
visualization is the
process of imagining

exactly what you want
to achieve or attain, and
also mentally rehearsing
what you'll need to do
to achieve or attain it.
Numerous largely
successful
individualities,
including celebrities,
have supported the use
of visualization,
claiming that it's played
a significant part in their
success. similar stars
include Bill Gates,
Arnold
Schwarzenegger,
Anthony Robbins, Tiger
Woods, Will Smith, Jim
Carey, and yet again,
the one and only,
Oprah.(Hmm could
there be a link between
Oprah being one of the
successful women in the
world, and the fact that
she practices most, if
not all six of the Life

S.A.V.E.R.S.?) Tiger Woods, arguably the topmost golfer of all time, is notorious for using visualization to mentally rehearse impeccably prosecution of his golf swing on every hole. Another world champion golfer, Jack Nicklaus, has said "I no way hit a shot, not indeed in practice, without having a veritably sharp in- focus picture of it in my head." Will Smith stated that he used visualization to overcome challenges, and imaged his success times before actually getting successful. Another notorious illustration is actor Jim Carrey, who wrote himself a check in 1987 in the quantum of 10 million bones. He dated it for "Thanksgiving 1995" and added in the memo line, "For acting services rendered." He also imaged it four times, and in 1994 he was paid 10 million for his starring part in Dumb and Dumber.

Utmost people are limited by fancies of their history, replaying former failures and dolor. Creative Visualization enables you to design the vision that will enthrall your mind, icing that the topmost pull on you is your future a compelling, instigative, and measureless future. There's a brief summary of how I use Visualization, followed by three simple ways for you to produce your own Visualization process. After I've read my declarations, I sit upright on my living room settee, close my eyes, and take a many slow, deep breaths. For the coming five twinkles, I simply fantasize myself living my ideal day, performing all of my tasks with ease, confidence, and enjoyment. For illustration, during the months that I spent writing this book (okay, who am I kidding it took times), I would first fantasize myself writing with ease, enjoying the creative process, free from stress, fear, and pen's block. I also imaged the end result people reading the finished book, loving it and telling their musketeers about it. Imaging the process being pleasurable, free from stress and fear, motivated me to take action and overcome procrastination.

Three Simple ways For Miracle Morning Visualization

Directly after reading your declarations where you took the time to articulate and concentrate on your pretensions and who you need to be to take your life to the coming position is the high time to fantasize yourself living in alignment with your declarations. Step 1 Get Ready Some people like to play necessary music in the background similar as classical or baroque (check out anything from the musician Bach) during their visualization. However, put it on with the volume fairly low, if you'd like to experiment with playing music. Now, sit up altitudinous, in a comfortable position. This can be on a president, settee, bottom, etc. Breathe deeply. Close your eyes, clear your mind, and get ready to fantasize. Step 2 fantasizes What You Really Want numerous people do not feel comfortable imaging success and are indeed spooked to succeed. Some people may witness resistance in this area. Some may indeed feel shamefaced that they will leave the other 95 behind when they come successful. This notorious quotation from Marianne Williamson's bestselling book, A Return To Love, may reverberate with anyone who feels internal or emotional obstacles when trying to fantasize " Our deepest fear isn't that we're shy. Our deepest fear is that we're   important beyond measure. It's our light, not our darkness that utmost frightens us. We ask ourselves, who am I to be brilliant, gorgeous, talented, and fabulous? Actually, who are you not to be? You're a child   of God. You're playing small

doesn't serve the world.
There's nothing
enlightened about
shrinking so that other
people won't feel
insecure around you.
We're all meant to
shine, as children do.
We were born to make
overload the glory of
God that's within us. It's
not just in some of us;
it's in everyone. And as
we let our own light
shine, we unconsciously
give other people
authorization to do the
same. As we're
delivered from our own
fear, our presence
automatically liberates
others. " The topmost
gift we can give to the
people we love is to live
to our full eventuality.
What does that look like
for you? What do you
really want? Forget

about sense, limits, and being practical. However, do anything you wanted, and be anything you wanted, what would you have? What would you do? What would you be? If you could have anything you wanted. Visualize your major pretensions, deepest solicitations, and utmost instigative, would- completely- change- my- life- if- I- achieved- them dreams. See, feel, hear, touch, taste, and smell every detail of your vision. Involve all of your senses to maximize the effectiveness of your visualization. The more pictorial you make your vision, the more compelled you'll be to take the necessary conduct to make it a reality. Now, forward into the future to see yourself achieving your ideal issues and results. You can either look towards the near unborn the end of the day or further into the future, like I did while writing this book, when I imaged people reading it, loving it, and recommending it to their musketeers. The point is you want to see yourself negotiating what you set out to negotiate, and you want to experience how good it'll feel to have followed through and achieved your pretensions. Step 3 fantasize Who You Need To Be and What You Need To Do Once you 've created a clear internal picture of what you want, begin to fantasize yourself living in total alignment with the person you need to be to achieve your vision. See yourself engaged in the positive conduct you'll need to do each day (exercising, studying, working, writing, making calls, transferring emails, etc.) and make sure you see yourself enjoying the process. See yourself smiling as you're running on that routine, filled with a sense of pride for your tone-discipline to follow through. Picture the look of determination on your face as you confidently, persistently make those phone calls, work on that report, or eventually take action and make progress on

that design you 've
been putting off for far
too long. Fantasize your
co-workers, guests,
family, musketeers, and
partner responding to
your positive address
and auspicious outlook.

Final Studies on Visualization

In addition to reading
your declarations every
morning, doing this
simple visualization
process every day will
turbo- charge the
programming of your
subconscious mind for
success. You'll begin to
live in alignment with
your ideal vision and
make it a reality.
Imaging your
pretensions and dreams
is believed by some
experts to attract your

fancies into your life.
Whether or not you
believe in the law of
magnet, there are
practical operations for
visualization. When
you fantasize what you
want, you stir up
feelings that lift your
spirits and pull you
towards your vision.
The more vividly you
see what you want, and
the more intensively
you allow yourself to
experience now the
passions you'll feel once
you 've achieved your
thing, the more you
make the possibility of
achieving it feel real.
When you fantasize
daily, you align your
studies and passions
with your vision. This
makes it easier to
maintain the
provocation you need to

continue taking the necessary conduct. Visualization can be an important aid to prostrating tone-limiting habits similar as procrastination, and to taking the conduct necessary to achieve your pretensions. I recommend starting with just five twinkles of visualization. still, in the coming chapter The 6- nanosecond phenomenon Morning I 'm going to educate you how you can gain the important benefits of imaging in just one nanosecond per day.

Vision Boards were made popular by the bestselling book and film The Secret. A Vision Board is simply a bill board on which you post images of what you want to have, who you want to come, what you want to do, where you want to live, etc. Creating a Vision Board is a fun exertion you can do on your own, with a friend, your significant other, or indeed your kiddies. It gives you commodity palpable to concentrate on during your Visualization. If you'd like detailed instructions on this process, Christine Kane has an excellent blog on How to Make a Vision Board as well as a free eBook named The Complete companion To Vision Boards. Keep in mind that, although creating a Vision Board is delightful, nothing changes in your life without action. I've to agree with Neil Farber, M.D., Ph.D., who stated in his composition on.psychologytoday.com, "Vision boards are for featuring, action boards are for achieving." While looking at your vision board every day may increase your provocation and help you stay focused on your pretensions, know that only taking the necessary conduct will get you real- time results.

Morning exercise should be a chief in your diurnal rituals. When you exercise for indeed a many twinkles every morning it significantly boosts your energy, enhances your health, improves tone-confidence and emotional well- being, and enables you to suppose better and concentrate longer. Too busy for exercise? In the coming chapter, I'll show you how to fit in a drill every day in as little as 60 seconds. I lately saw an eye-opening videotape with particular development expert and tone- made multi-millionaire entrepreneur, Eben Pagan, who was being canvassed by bestselling author Anthony Robbins. Tony asked, "Eben, what's your #1 key to success?" Of course, I was veritably encouraged when Eben's response was, "Start every morning off with a particular success ritual. That's the most important key to success. " also he went on to talk about the significance of morning exercise. Eben said, "Every morning, you've got to get your heart rate up and get your blood flowing and fill your lungs with oxygen. "He continued, "Don't just exercise at the end of the day or at the middle of the day. And indeed if you do like to exercise at those times, always incorporate at least 10 to 20 twinkles of jumping jacks or some kind of aerobic exercise in the morning. " The benefits of morning exercise are too numerous to ignore. From waking you up and enhancing your internal clarity, to helping you sustain advanced situations of energy throughout the day, exercising soon after rising can ameliorate your life in numerous ways. Whether you go to the spa, go for a walk or run, throw on a P90XTM or Insanity TM DVD, what you do during your period of exercise is over to you, although I'll share some recommendations. Tête-à-tête, if I were only allowed to exercise one form of exercise for the rest of my life, I would, without mistrustfulness choose yoga. I began rehearsing yoga shortly after I created The Miracle Morning, and have been doing it and loving it ever ago. It's such a complete form of

exercise, as it combines
stretching with strength
training with cardio
with focused breathing,
and can indeed be a
form of contemplation.
Meet the One and Only
Dashama I can't talk
about yoga (or exercise
for that matter) without
talking about my friend
Dashama. A many times
ago, one of her
scholars introduced me
to her work as one of
the world's leading
yoga   preceptors.
Dashama is the most
authentic, spiritual,
practical, and   each-
around most effective
yoga schoolteacher I've
ever come through. I
asked her to partake her
unique perspective on
the benefits of yoga.
The important thing to
remember is that yoga

can take place in many forms. Whether it is sitting in silent meditation, breathing to expand your lung capacity or back bending to open your heart - there are practices that can help every aspect of your life. The key is to learn which techniques to practice when you need a remedy and use it to your advantage to bring yourself into balance. A well-rounded yoga practice can enhance your life in so many ways. It can heal what is out of harmony and can move stuck or blocked energy through your body, creating space for new fluid movement, blood flow and energy to circulate. I encourage you to listen to your body and try some new sequences as you feel ready.

Final Studies On Exercise

You know that if you want to maintain good health and increase your energy, you must exercise constantly. That's not news to anybody. But it's too easy to make defenses as to why we don't exercise. Two of the biggest are "I just don't have time "and "I 'm just too tired." There's no limit to the defenses that you can suppose of. The more creative you're the further defenses you can come up with, right? That's the beauty of incorporating exercise into your phenomenon Morning; it happens before your day wears you out, before you have a chance to get too tired, before you have an entire day to come up with new defenses for avoiding exercise. The Miracle Morning is really a surefire way to avoid all of those defenses, and to make exercise a daily habit.(further on the easy way to apply positive habits into your life, like exercise, in Chapter 9 From unsupportable To impregnable- The Real Secret To Forming Habits That Will transfigure Your Life(In 30 Days) which will enhance your quality of life for times to come.)

Reading, the fifth practice in the Life S.A.V.E.R.S., is the fast track to transubstantiating any area of your life. It's one of the most immediate styles for acquiring the knowledge, ideas, and strategies you need to achieve Level 10 success in any area of your life. The key is to learn from the experts those who have formerly done what you want to do. Don't resuscitate the wheel. The fastest way to achieve everything you want is to model successful people who have formerly achieved it. With an nearly horizon less quantum of

books available on
every content, there are
no limits to the
knowledge you can gain
through diurnal reading.
I lately heard someone
say in a mocking, I 'm
too cool for this tone,
"Uh, yeah, I don't read
'tone- help' books," as
if similar books were
beneath him. Poor Joe. I
'm not sure if it's his
pride or just lack of
mindfulness, but he's
missing out on the
unlimited force of
knowledge, bottomless
growth and life
changing ideas he could
gain from some of the
most brilliant,
successful
individualities in the
world. Who in their
right mind would
choose not to do that?
Whatever you want for

your life, there are innumerous books on how to get it. Want to come fat, rich, a multi-millionaire? There are plenitude of books written by those who have achieved the pinnacles of fiscal success which will educate you how. Then are a many of my pets suppose and Grow Rich by Napoleon Hill Secrets of the Millionaire Mind by T. Harv Eker Total Money Makeover by Dave Ramsey Want to produce an inconceivable, loving, probative and romantic relationship? There are presumably more books on how to do exactly that than you could read in a decade. Then are a many of my pets The

Five Love Languages
by Gary D. Chapman
the Soul Mate
Experience by Jo Dunn
the Seven Principles for
Making a Marriage
Work by John M.
Gottman and Nan Silver
Whether you 'd like to
transfigure your
connections, increase
your tone- confidence,
ameliorate your
communication or
persuasion chops, learn
how to come fat, or
ameliorate any area of
your life, head to your
original bookstore or do
what I do and head to
Amazon.com and you
'll find a plethora of
books on any area of
your life you want to
ameliorate.

**How Important
Should You Read?**

I recommend making a commitment to read a minimum of 10 runners per day (although five is okay to start with, if you read sluggishly or don't yet enjoy reading). Let's do some calculation on this for an alternate reading 10 runners read per day isn't going to break you, but it'll make you. We're only talking 10- 15 twinkles of reading or 15- 30 twinkles if you read more sluggishly. Look at it this way. However, reading just 10 runners a day will average 3, 650 runners a time, If you quantify that. Final studies On Reading Begin with the end in mind. Before you begin reading each day, ask yourself why you're reading that book what you want to gain from it and keep that outgrowth in mind. Take a moment to do this now by asking yourself what you want to gain from reading this book. Are you committed to finishing it? More importantly, are you committed to enforcing what you 're literacy and taking action, by following through with The Miracle Morning 30-Day Life Transformation Challenge at the end? Numerous phenomenon Morning interpreters use their Reading time to catch up on their religious textbooks, similar as the Bible, Torah, or any other. Hopefully you took the advice I gave and you 've been italicizing, circling, pressing, folding the corners of runners, and taking notes in the perimeters of this book. To get the most out of any book I read and make it easy for me to readdress the content again in the future, I accentuate or circle anything that I may want tore-visit, and make notes in the perimeters to remind me why I underscored that particular section.(Unless, of course, it's a library book). This process of marking books as I read allows me to come back at any time and regain all of the crucial assignments, ideas, and benefits without demanding to read the book again, cover to cover. I largely

recommend re-reading
good particular
development books.
Infrequently can we
read a book formerly
and internalize all of the
value from that book.
Achieving mastery in
any area requires
reiteration being
exposed to certain ideas,
strategies, or ways over
and over again, until
they come engrained in
your subconscious
mind. For illustration, if
you wanted to master
karate, you would not
learn the ways formerly
and also suppose, "I got
this." No, you'd learn
the ways, exercise them,
also go back to your
sensei and learn them
again, and repeat the
process hundreds of
times in order to master
a single fashion.

Learning ways to ameliorate your life works the same way. There's further value in re-reading a book you formerly know has strategies that can ameliorate your life than there is in reading a new book before you've learned the strategies in the first. Whenever I 'm reading a book that I see can really make an impact on an area of my life, I commit tore-reading that book(or at least-reading the corridor I 've underscored, circled and stressed) as soon as I 'm finished going through it the first time. I actually keep a special space on my bookshelf for the books that I want tore-read. I've read books like suppose and

Grow Rich as numerous as three times, and frequently relate back to them throughout the time. Re-reading requires discipline, because it's generally more "fun" to read a book you've no way read ahead. Repetition can be that's indeed more reason why we should do it to develop an advanced boring or tedious (which is why so many people ever "master" anything), but position of tone-discipline. Why not try it out with this book? Commit tore-reading it as soon as you 're finished, to consolidate your literacy and give yourself more   time to master The Miracle Morning.

Seaming is the final practice in the Life S.A.V.E.R.S. and is really just another word for jotting, but please allow me to keep it real I demanded an ' S ' for the end of Life S.A.V.E.R.S. because a ' W ' would not fit anywhere. Thanks Thesaurus, I owe you one. Journaling My favorite form of Scribing is journaling, which I do for 5- 10 twinkles during my Miracle Morning. By getting your studies out of your head and putting them in jotting, you gain precious perceptivity you'd else no way see. The seaming element of your Miracle Morning enables you to validate your perceptivity, ideas, improvements, consummations, successes, and assignments learned, as well as any areas of occasion, particular growth, or enhancement. While I had known about the profound benefits of journaling for times and I had indeed tried it a many times I no way stuck with it constantly, because it was no way part of my diurnal routine. generally, I kept a journal by my bed, and when I 'd get home late at night, nine times out of ten I would find myself making the reason that I was too tired to write in it. My journals stayed substantially blank. Indeed though I formerly had numerous substantially blank journals sitting on my bookshelf, every so frequently I would buy myself a brand new journal a more precious one persuading myself that if I spent a lot of plutocrat on it, I would surely write in it. Seems like a decent proposition, right? Unfortunately, my little strategy no way worked, and for times I just accumulated more and more decreasingly precious, yet inversely empty journals. That was before The Miracle Morning. From day one, The Miracle Morning gave me the time and structure to write in my journal every day, and it snappily came one of my favorite habits. I can tell you now that journaling has come one

of the most comforting
and fulfilling practices
of my life. Not only do I
decide the diurnal
benefits of purposely
directing my studies
and putting them in
jotting, but indeed more
important are those I've
gained from reviewing
my journals, from cover
to cover, latterly
especially, at the end of
the time. It is hard to put
into words how
overwhelmingly
formative the
experience of going
back and reviewing
your journals can be,
but I'll do my stylish.
My First Journal Re-
view On December
31st, after my first time
doing The phenomenon
Morning and jotting in
my journal, I began
reading the first runner

I had written that time.
Day by day, I started to
review and relive my
entire time. I was
suitable to readdress my
mindset from each day,
and gain a new
perspective as to how
important I had grown
throughout the time. I
redefined my conduct,
conditioning, and
progress, giving me a
new appreciation for
how important I had
fulfilled during the once
12 months. Most
importantly, I
reacquired the
assignments I had
learned, numerous of
which I had forgotten
over the course of the
time. Gratitude2.0 I
also endured a
important deeper quality
of gratefulness in a
way that I had no way

endured before on two different situations, contemporaneously. It was what I now relate to as my first Back to the unborn moment. Try to follow me then (and feel free to picture me as Marty McFly stepping out of a 1985 DeLorean). As I read through my journal, my current tone(which was also the future   tone of who I was at the time I wrote those journal entries) was now looking back at all of the people, gests , assignments, and accomplishments that I took note of being thankful for throughout the time. As I was in that moment reliving the gratefulness that I felt in the   history, I was contemporaneously

feeling thankful in the
present moment for
how far I had come
since that time in my
life. It was a remarkable
experience, and a bit
surreal. Accelerated
Growth- also, I began to
tap into the loftiest point
of value I would gain
from reviewing my
journals. I pulled out a
distance of blank paper,
drew a line down the
middle, and wrote two
headlines at the top
Assignments Learned
and New Commitments.
As I read through my
hundreds of my journal
entries, I set up myself
retrieving dozens of
precious assignments.
This process of
retrieving Assignments
Learned and making
New Commitments to
apply those assignments

backed my particular growth and development further than nearly anything differently. While there are numerous worthwhile benefits of keeping a diurnal journal, a many of which I 've just described, then are a many further of my pets § Gain Clarity- The process of writing commodity down forces us to suppose through it enough to understand it. Journaling will give you further clarity, allow you to communicate, and help you work through problems. Capture Ideas- Journaling helps you not only expand your ideas, but also prevent you from losing the important ideas that you may want to act on in the future. Review Assignments- It enables you to review all of the assignments you've learned. Admit Your Progress- It's awful to go back andre-read your journal entries from a time ago and see how important progress you've made. It's one of the most empowering, confidence- inspiring and pleasurable gests. It can't really be duplicated any other way. Gap- Focus Is It Hurting or Helping You? In the opening runners of this chapter, we talked about using the Life S.A.V.E.R.S. to close your " Implicit Gap. " mortal beings are conditioned to have what I call Gap- focus. We tend to concentrate

on the gaps between
where we're in life and
where we want to be,
between what we 've
accomplished and what
we could have or want
to negotiate, and the
gap between who we're
and our romantic vision
of the person we believe
we should be. The
problem with this is that
constant Gap- focus can
be mischievous to our
confidence and tone-
image, causing us to
feel like we do not have
enough, have not
fulfilled enough, and
that we're simply not
good enough, or at least,
not as good as we
should be. High
achievers are generally
the worst at this,
constantly overlooking
or minimizing their
accomplishments,

beating themselves up over every mistake and fault, and no way is feeling like anything they do relatively good enough. The irony is that gap- focus is a big part of the reason that high achievers are high achievers. Their inextinguishable desire to close the gap is what energies their pursuit of excellence and constantly drives them to   achieve. Gap- focus can be healthy and productive if it comes from a positive, visionary, "I 'm committed to and agitated about fulfilling my eventuality" perspective, without any passions of lack. Unfortunately, it infrequently does. The average person, indeed the average high achiever, tends to concentrate negatively on their gaps. The loftiest achievers those who are balanced and concentrated on achieving Level 10 success in nearly every area of their lives are exceedingly thankful for what they have, regularly admit themselves for what they 've fulfilled, and are always at peace with where they're in their lives. It's the battering idea that I'm doing the stylish that I can in this moment, and at the same time, I can and will do better. This balanced tone-assessment prevents that feeling of lack of not being, having, doing enough while still

allowing them to
constantly strive to
close their implicit gap
in each area. Generally,
when a day, week,
month, or time ends,
and we're in Gap- focus
mode, it's nearly
insolvable to maintain
an accurate assessment
of ourselves and our
progress. For
illustration, if you had
10 effects on your to-
do list for the day
indeed if you completed
six of them your Gap-
focus causes you to feel
you did not get
everything done that
you wanted to do. The
maturity of people does
dozens, indeed
hundreds, of effects
right during the day, and
a many effects wrong.
Guess which effects
people flash back and

renewal in their minds over and over again? Does not make further sense to concentrate on the 100 that affects you right? It sure is more pleasurable. What does this have to do with jotting in a journal? Writing in a journal each day, with a structured, strategic process(more on that in a nanosecond) allows you to direct your focus to what you did negotiate, what you 're thankful for, and what you 're committed to doing better hereafter. Therefore, you more deeply enjoy your trip each day, feel good about any forward progress you made, and use a heightened position of clarity to accelerate your results.

Final Studies On The Life S.A.V.E.R.S.

Everything is delicate before it's easy. Every new experience is uncomfortable before it's comfortable. The more you exercise the Life the more natural and normal each of them will feel. Flash back that my first time planning was nearly my last, as my mind contended like a Ferrari and my studies bounced around uncontrollably like the tableware sphere in a pinball machine. Now, I love contemplation, and while I 'm no master, I'd say I 'm decent at it. Also, my first time doing yoga, I felt like a fish out of water. I was not flexible, could not do the acts rightly, and felt awkward and uncomfortable. Now, yoga is my favorite form of exercise, and I'm so thankful that I stuck with it. I invite you to begin rehearsing the Life S.A.V.E.R.S. Now, so you can come familiar and comfortable with each of them, and get a jump-launch before you begin The Miracle Morning 30 Day Life Transformation Challenge in Chapter 10. If your biggest concern is still chancing time, don't worry, I've got you covered. In the coming chapter, you're going to learn how to do the entire Miracle Morning entering the full benefits from all six

of the Life S.A.V.E.R.S.
in only 6 twinkles a day.

CHAPTER SEVEN

The busy person's 6-minute miracle

Oh, you're busy?
Weird. I allowed it, was
just me. Presumably the
most common question
or concern I get about
The Miracle Morning is
regarding how long it
needs to be. When I first
had the advance
consummation about
how our situations of
success(and fulfilling
our eventuality) in
every area of life are
being limited by our
inadequate(or missing)
position of particular
development, my

biggest challenge was chancing time to act on this consummation. As I've developed and participated The Miracle Morning over the times, I've been veritably apprehensive of the need to make it scalable so that indeed the busiest among us can make time for our Miracle Morning. I developed The 6-nanosecond phenomenon Morning for those days when you're redundant busy and pressed for time, as well as for those of you who are so overwhelmed with your life situation right now that just allowing about adding one further thing stresses you out. I suppose we can each agree that investing a

minimum of six
twinkles into getting
the person we need to
be to produce the
situations of success
and happiness we truly
want in our lives isn't
only reasonable, it's an
absolute must-have,
indeed when we 're
pressed for time. I
suppose you'll be
pleasantly surprised in
the coming many
twinkles as you read and
realize how important
(and life- changing)
these six twinkles can
be! Imagine if the first
six twinkles of every
morning began like this
Minute One fantasize
yourself waking up
peacefully in the
morning, with a big
nudnik , a stretch, and a
smile on your face.
Rather of rushing

carelessly into your excited day stressed and overwhelmed you spend the first nanosecond sitting still, in purposeful Silence. You sit, veritably calm, veritably peaceful, and breathe deeply, sluggishly. Perhaps you say a prayer of gratefulness to appreciate the moment, or supplicate for guidance on your trip. Perhaps you decide to try your first nanosecond of contemplation. As you sit in silence, you're completely present in the now, in the moment. You calm your mind, relax your body, and allow all of your stress to melt down. You develop a deeper sense of peace, purpose, and

direction Minute Two
You pull out your
diurnal declarations the
bones that remind you
of your unlimited
eventuality and you're
most important
precedence and you
read them out loud from
top to bottom. As you
concentrate on what's
most important to you,
your position of internal
provocation increases.
Reading over the
monuments of how able
you really are gives you
a feeling of confidence.
Looking over what
you're committed to,
what your purpose is,
and what your
pretensions are re-
energizes you to take
the   conduct necessary
to live the life you truly
want, earn, and now
know is possible for you

Minute Three You close your eyes, or you look at your vision board and you   fantasize. Your Visualization could include what it'll look and feel like when you reach your pretensions. You fantasize the day going   impeccably, see yourself enjoying your work, smiling and laughing with your family or your significant other, and fluently negotiating all that you intend to negotiate for that day. You see what it'll look like, you feel what it'll feel like, and you witness the joy of what you will produce

Minute Four You take one nanosecond to write down some of the effects that you 're thankful for, what you 're proud of, and the results you 're committed to creating for that day. In doing so, you produce for yourself an empowered, inspired, and confident state of mind Minute Five also; you snare your tone- help book and invest one miraculous nanosecond reading a runner or two. You learn a new idea, commodity you can incorporate into your day which will ameliorate your results at work or in your connections. You discover commodity new that you can use to suppose and feel more to live more Minute Six Eventually; you stand up and spend the last nanosecond moving your body for 60 seconds. Perhaps you run in place, perhaps you do a nanosecond of jumping- jacks. Perhaps you do push- ups or sit- ups. The point is that you're getting your heart rate over, generating energy and adding your capability to be alert and focused. How would you feel if that's how you employed the first 6- twinkles of each day? How would the quality of your day your life ameliorates? I do not suggest you limit your phenomenon Morning to only six twinkles every day, but as I said, on those days when you're pressed for time, The 6- nanosecond phenomenon Morning provides an important strategy for accelerating

your particular
development.

CHAPTER EIGHT

Customizing your
Miracle Morning
routine

Up until this point,
we've primarily been
concentrated on the Life
S.A.V.E.R.S. model to
accelerate your
particular development
during your Miracle
Morning. Still, The
Miracle Morning is 100
customizable.
Everything from your
wake- up time to the
total duration of your
Miracle Morning to
which conditioning you

do, as well as the duration and order of each exertion there is no limit to how your Miracle Morning can be substantiated to fit your life and help you achieve your most significant pretensions, faster than ever ahead. Then I'll cover all of the below, as well as when (and what) to eat in the morning, how to align The Miracle Morning with your major pretensions and dreams, what to do on the weekends, a tip on prostrating procrastination, and much further. Wake Up and Start Time This may sound fully untoward intuitive, but stick with me. You do not actually have to do The Miracle Morning in the morning. Huh? Of course there are inarguable advantages to beforehand rising and getting a visionary launch to your day. Still, for some, their unique schedule and life simply may not allow it. Obviously, someone who works the graveyard shift, or indeed late- nights, is going to have a different wake up time than someone who's in bed by 900p.m. every evening. Considering that different people have different schedules, the substance of The Miracle Morning remains that you simply wake up earlier than you typically would(generally by 30- 60 twinkles), so that you can devote time every day to perfecting yourself, so you can transfigure your life. When, Why, and what to Eat (In the Morning) Up until this point, you may have been wondering when the heck do I get to eat during my Miracle Morning?! I'll cover that then. Besides when you eat during your Miracle Morning, what you choose to eat is indeed more critical, and why you choose to eat what you eat may be most important of all. When To Eat- Keep in mind that digesting food is one of the most energy- draining processes the body goes through each day. The bigger the mess, the further food you give your body to condensation, the further drained you'll feel. With that in mind, I recommend eating after your Miracle Morning. This ensures that, for optimum alertness and focus during the Life S.A.V.E.R.S., your blood will be flowing to your brain rather than to your stomach to digest your food. Still, make sure that it's a small, light, if you feel like you must eat commodity first thing in the morning. Why To Eat- Let's take a moment to bandy why you eat the   foods that you do. When you're shopping at the grocery store, or opting food from a menu at an eatery, what criteria do you use to determine which foods you're going to put into your body? Are your choices grounded purely on taste? Texture? Convenience? Are they grounded on health? Energy? Salutary restrictions? utmost people eat the foods they do grounded substantially on the taste, and at a deeper position, grounded on our emotional attachment to the foods we like the taste .However, " Why did you eat that ice cream? Why did you drink that soda pop? " Or, "Why did you bring that fried funk home from the grocery store?" You would most probably hear responses like, if you were to ask someone. I was in the

mood for fried funk. ”
All answers grounded
on the emotional
enjoyment deduced
primarily from the way
these foods taste. In this
case, this person isn't
likely to explain their
food choices with how
important value these
foods will add to their
health, or how important
sustained energy they’ll
get. My point is this If
we want to have further
energy(which we all
do) and if we want our
lives to be healthy and
complaint-free(which
we all do) also it’s
pivotal that we
reevaluate why we eat
the foods that we do,
and this is important
launch valuing the
health benefits and
energy consequences of
the foods we eat as

important as or further than the taste. In no way am I saying that we should eat foods that do not taste good in exchange for the health and energy benefits. I 'm saying that we can have both. I 'm saying that if we want to live every day with an cornucopia of energy so we can perform at our stylish and live a long, healthy life, we must choose to eat further foods that are good for our health and give us sustained energy, as well as tasting great. What to Eat- Before we talk about what to eat, let's take a second to talk about what to drink. Flash back that Step# 4 of the 5- Step Snooze-evidence Wake up Strategy is to drink a full glass of water   first thing in the morning so you can desiccate and reenergize   after a full night of sleep. Next, I generally start my Miracle Morning by brewing a mug of high quality tea. I actually set my alarm 15 twinkles before each day, to give myself time to make my tea without intruding on my Miracle Morning time. However, feel free to brew your favorite mug of coffee, if you're a coffee toper. As for what to eat, it has been proven that a diet rich in living foods, similar as fresh fruits and vegetables will greatly increase your energy situations, ameliorate your internal focus and emotional wellbeing, keep you healthy, and

cover you from
complaint. So, I created
the phenomenon
Morning Super-food
Smoothie that
incorporates everything
your body needs in one
altitudinous, frosty
glass! I 'm talking about
complete protein(all of
the essential amino
acids), age defying
antioxidants, Omega 3
Essential Adipose
Acids(to boost
impunity,
cardiovascular health,
and brain power), plus a
rich diapason of
vitamins and minerals
and that's just for
starters. I have not
indeed mentioned all
the super-foods, similar
as the stimulating,
mood- lifting
phytonutrients in
Cacao(the tropical bean

from which chocolate is made), the long- lasting energy of Maca (the Andean adaptogen deified for its hormone-balancing goods), and the vulnerable- boosting nutrients and appetite-suppressing parcels of Chia seeds. The Miracle Morning Super-food Smoothie not only provides you with sustained energy, it also tastes great. You might indeed find that it enhances your capability to produce cautions in your everyday life. Flash back the old saying you're what you eat? Take care of your body so your body will take care of you. You'll feel vibrant energy and enhanced clarity incontinently! Aligning

The Miracle Morning
with Your pretensions
& utmost phenomenon
Morning interpreters
and high achievers use
The Miracle Morning to
enhance their focus on
their immediate
pretensions and their
most significant dreams.
This is especially true
for those they've been
putting off, or have not
been making time for
similar as starting a
business or writing a
book. The Life
S.A.V.E.R.S. is ideal for
perfecting your
capability to stay
focused on your
pretensions and
accelerating the rate at
which you make
progress towards your
dreams. For illustration,
when you produce your
declarations, make sure

that they're in alignment
with your pretensions
and dreams, and that
they clarify what you'll
need to suppose,
believe, and do to
achieve them, so they
support your unvarying
commitment to follow
through. Reading them
daily will keep you
concentrated on your
loftiest precedence and
the way you need to
take to achieve them.
When you are doing
your morning
Visualization, fantasize
yourself painlessly
enjoying the process of
achieving your
pretensions (like I did
while writing this book)
and keep a clear picture
of what it'll look like
formerly achieved.
Flash back to involve all
of your senses, see, feel,

taste, touch and indeed smell every detail of your vision and your ideal issues. The more pictorial your vision is, the more effective it'll be in adding your desire and provocation to take the necessary way towards your pretensions each day. Prostrating procrastination Do the Worst, First One of the most effective strategies for prostrating habitual procrastination and maximizing your productivity is to start working on your most important or least pleasurable tasks, first thing in the morning. In his bestselling book Eat That Frog, the fabulous productivity expert Brian Tracy shows how getting effects done in

the morning leads to
internal prices that can
take us to great heights
in our lives. It's the idea
that doing the hard task
first(" frog eating ")
and getting   it out of
the way creates
instigation and makes
the rest of the day more
productive. The
purpose of The Miracle
Morning is further
about waking up with
purpose combining the
benefits of early rising
and particular
development and is not
so much concerned with
which conditioning you
do, as long as the
conditioning you choose
are visionary and help
you ameliorate your
inner world(yourself)
and your external
world(your life). In
this short chapter I'll

give you some ideas and strategies for how you can design your Miracle Morning and acclimate it to fit your life so it adds value to your life and helps you achieve your most important pretensions. I 'll also include exemplifications of different real- life phenomenon Mornings, designed by individualities from entrepreneurs to stay- at- home mothers, to high academy and council scholars to fit their unique schedules, precedence and cultures. The phenomenon Morning on Weekends "Waking up beforehand on Saturday gives me an edge in finishing my work with a veritably relaxed state of mind. There's a feeling of time pressure on weekdays that are not there on weekends. However, before anybody differently, I can plan the day or at least my conditioning with relaxed mind, if I wake up beforehand in the morning. " Oprah Winfrey I could not agree with Oprah more. When I first created The Miracle Morning I only did it Monday through Friday, and I took the weekends off. It did not take long for me to realize that every day I did The Miracle Morning I felt better, more fulfilled and more productive, but every day that I slept in, I woke feeling sleepy, unfocused, and unproductive. You may start, as I did, by doing the phenomenon Morning during the week and try taking the weekends off. See how you feel on those Saturday and Sunday mornings, sleeping, like numerous people do, that every day is better when you begin it with The Miracle Morning, if you feel. Keeping Your Miracle Morning Fresh, Fun, and instigative! Over the times, my Miracle Morning continues to evolve. While I still exercise the Life S.A.V.E.R.S. daily and do not prevision any reason I would ever stop demanding the benefits of those six practices, I do suppose it's important to mix effects up and keep variety in

your Miracle Morning.
Like a relationship, you
always want to keep a
little fun and excitement
in the blend, so effects
do not get boring or
banal. For illustration,
you might change up
your morning exercise
routine every 90 days,
or indeed yearly. You
could try different
contemplations, either
through a simple
Google hunt or by
downloading colorful
Meditation apps on your
phone. You could
produce a vision board
and modernize it
regularly. As I
mentioned during the
section on declarations
you should always be
streamlining your
declarations to stimulate
your senses and to be in
alignment with your

always- evolving vision
for who you can and
want to be.

CHAPTER NINE

From unbearable to
unstoppable – the real
secret 30 days

It's been said that our
quality of life is created
by the quality of our
habits. However, also
that person simply has
the habits in place that
are creating and
sustaining their

situations of success, if a person is living a successful life. On the other hand, if someone isn't passing the situations of success they want no matter what the area they simply have not committed to putting the necessary habits in place which will produce the results they want. Considering that our habits produce our life, there's arguably no single skill that's more important for you to learn and master than controlling your habits. You must identify, apply, and maintain the habits necessary for creating the results you want in your life, while learning how to let go of any negative habits which are holding you back from achieving your true eventuality. Habits are actions that are repeated regularly and tend to do subconsciously. Whether you realize it or not, your life has been, and will continue to be, created by your habits. However, your habits will control you, If you do not control your habits. Unfortunately, if you 're like the rest of us, you were no way tutored how to successfully apply and sustain(aka " master ") positive habits. There's no class offered in academy called Habit Mastery. There should be. Such a course would presumably be more important to your success and overall quality of life than all of the other courses combined. Because they no way learned to master their habits, utmost people fail at nearly every attempt to control them, time and time again. Take New Year's judgments, for illustration. Habitual Failure New Year's judgments (NYRs) Every time, millions of well- intentioned people make New Year's judgments, but lower than five percent of us stick to them. A NYR is really just a positive habit (like exercising or beforehand rising) you want to incorporate into your life, or a negative habit (like smoking or eating fast food) you want to get relieve of. You do not need a

statistic to tell you that,
when it comes to NYRs,
utmost people have
formerly given over and
thrown in the kerchief
before January has
indeed come to a close.
Perhaps you've seen
this miracle in real-time.
However, you know
how delicate it can be to
find a parking spot, if
you've ever gone to the
spa the first week of
January. It's packed
with vehicles possessed
by people with good
intentions, and armed
with a NYR to lose
weight and get in shape.
Still, if you go back to
the spa closer to the end
of the month, you'll
notice that half of the
parking lot is empty.
Not fortified with a
proven strategy to stick
with their new habits,

the maturity continues
to fail. Why is it so
delicate to apply and
sustain the habits we
need to be happy,
healthy, and successful?
Addicted to the Old
Change Is Painful Yes,
we are, at some
position, addicted to our
habits. Whether
psychologically or
physically, once a habit
has been corroborated
through enough
reiteration, it can be
veritably delicate to
change. That is, if you
do not have an effective,
proven strategy. One of
the primary reasons
utmost people fail to
produce and sustain new
habits is because they
do not knowing what to
anticipate, and they do
not have a winning
strategy. How Long

Does It Really Take To Form A New Habit? Depending on the composition you read or which expert you hear to, you 'll hear compelling substantiation that it takes anywhere from a single hypnotism session, 21 days, or indeed up to three months to incorporate a new habit into your life or get relieve of an old one. The popular 21-day myth may come from the 1960 book sickie- Cybernetics a New Way to get further Living out of Life. Written by ornamental surgeon Dr. Maxwell Maltz, he set up that amputees took, on average, 21 days to acclimate to the loss of a branch. He argued that people take 21 days to acclimate to any major life changes. Some would argue that how long it takes for a habit to come truly automatic also depends on the difficulty of the habit. My particular experience and the real-world results I 've seen working with hundreds of guiding guests has led me to the conclusion that you can change any habit in 30 days, if you have the right strategy. The problem is, utmost people do not have any strategy, let alone the right bone. So, time after time, they lose confidence in themselves and their capability to ameliorate, as failed attempt after failed attempt piles over and knocks them down. Commodity has to change. One of the biggest obstacles precluding utmost people from enforcing and sustaining positive habits is that they do not have the right strategy. They do not know what to anticipate and are not prepared to overcome the internal and emotional challenges that are part of the process of enforcing any new habit. We 'll start by dividing the 30- day time frame necessary to apply a positive new habit(or get relieve of an old, negative habit) into three 10- day phases. Each of these phases presents a different set of emotional challenges and internal roadblocks to sticking with the new habit. Since the average person isn't apprehensive of these challenges and roadblocks, when they face them, they give up because they do not know what to do to overcome them.

The first 10 days of enforcing any new habit, or clearing yourself of any old habit, can feel nearly unsupportable. Although the first many days can be easy and indeed instigative because it's commodity new as soon as the freshness wears off, reality sets in. You detest it. It's painful. It's not delightful presently. Every fiber of your being tends to repel and reject the change. Your mind rejects it and you suppose I detest this. Your body resists it and tells you I do not like how this feels. Still, now), during the first 10 days your experience might be commodity like this (The alarm timepiece sounds) Oh God, If your new habit is waking up beforehand (which might be a useful one to get started on. I 'm so tired. I need further sleep. Okay, just 10 further twinkles.(Hit snooze button) The problem for utmost people is that they do not realize that this putatively unsupportable first 10 days is only " temporary. " rather, they suppose it's the way the new habit feels, and will always feel, telling themselves If the new habit is this painful, forget it it's not worth it. As a result, 95 of our society the medium maturity fail, time and time again, to start exercise routines, quit smoking, ameliorate their diets, stick to a budget, or any other habit that would ameliorate their quality of life. That's where you have an advantage over the other 95. See, when you're set for these first 10 days, when you know that it is the price you pay for success, that the first 10 days will be grueling but they're also temporary, you can beat the odds and succeed! If the benefits are great enough, we can do anything for 10 days, right? So, the first 10 days of enforcing any new habit are not a   fun and games. You'll defy it. You might indeed detest it at times. But you can do it. Especially considering, it only gets easier from then, and the price is, oh just the capability to produce everything you want for your life. After you get through the first 10 days the most delicate 10 days you begin the 2nd 10- day phase, which is vastly easier.   You'll be getting used to your new habit. You'll also have developed some confidence and positive associations to the benefits of your habit. While days 11- 20 are not unsupportable, they are still uncomfortable and will bear discipline and commitment on your part. At this stage it'll still be tempting to fall back to your old actions. Representing the illustration of waking up beforehand as your new habit, it'll still be easier to sleep in because you've done it for so long. Stay married. You've formerly gone from unsupportable to Uncomfortable, and you're about to find out what it feels like to be impregnable.

When you enter the final 10 days the home stretch the many people that make it this far nearly always make a mischievous mistake clinging to the popular advice from the numerous experts who claim it only takes 21 days to form a new habit. Those experts are incompletely correct. It does take 21 days the first two phases to form a new habit. But the third 10- day phase is pivotal to sustaining your new habit, long term. The final 10 days is where you appreciatively support and associate pleasure with your new habit. You've been primarily associating pain and discomfort with it during the first 20 days. Rather of abhorring and defying your new habit, you start feeling proud of yourself for making it this far. Phase Three is also where the factual metamorphosis occurs,

as your new habit
becomes part of your
identity. It transcends
the space between
commodity you're
trying and who you're
getting. You start to see
yourself as someone
who lives the habit.
Back to our illustration
of waking up
beforehand you go from
having an identity that
says I'm not a "morning
person" to I'm a
morning person! Rather
of dreading your alarm
timepiece in the
morning, now when the
alarm goes off you're
agitated to wake up and
get going because
you've done it for over
20 days in a row.
You're starting to see
and feel the benefits.
Too numerous people
get exorbitantly

confident, stroke themselves on the back and suppose I 've done it for 20 days so I 'm just going to take as many days out. The problem is that those first twenty days are the most   grueling part of the process. Taking a many days out before you've invested the necessary time into appreciatively buttressing the habit makes it delicate to get back on. Its days 21- 30 where you really start enjoying the habit, which is what will make you continue it in the future. But I detest Running "I 'm not a runner however, Jon. In fact, I detest running. There's no way I could do it. " "Come on, Hal it's to raise plutocrat for the Front Row Foundation," Jon Berghoff responded. " Look, I did not suppose I could do a marathon either, but once you commit to it, you'll find a way to make it be. And I 'm telling you, it's truly a life changing experience! " "I'll suppose about it." Telling Jon I would suppose about it was really just my way of getting him off my reverse. Do not get me wrong, I absolutely believed in and supported the life-changing work done by the Front Row Foundation. I had been giving plutocrat to the association for times, but writing a check was a little easier than running a marathon.

Unless I was being chased, I had not designedly run so much as a block in the 10 times since I graduated high academy. And indeed back also I only ran to keep from failing PE class. Besides, ever since breaking my femur and pelvis in the auto accident, back when I was 20, I was always hysterical of what might be if I put too important pressure on my leg. In fact, every time I went snow skiing, I could not help but have fancies of me tripping and taking a hard fall, also having the essence rod in my leg break through the skin of my ham. It's a horrible study, but breaking your branches and being told you may no way walk again can do that to you. A week latterly after my discussion with Jon, one of my guiding guests Katie Fingerhut completed her alternate marathon. "Hal, it's so amazing I feel like I can do anything now!" Between Jon and Katie's enthusiastic testaments for marathon handling, I was starting to suppose perhaps it was time for me to overcome my limiting belief about not being a runner, and just start running. Like everything differently in life, if they could do it, also so could I. So I did. The coming morning, intent on completing my first afar on my trip to completing a marathon, I put on my basketball shoes (sound familiar?) and headed out the frontal door of my house. I was actually looking forward to it! (Flash back; the first many days of any new habit are frequently instigative.) Down the driveway I hustled, motivated and inspired. Onto the sidewalk I ran. As I stepped from the sidewalk to the road, my ankle twisted on the check and I collapsed. Lying on the pavement, writhing in pain and gripping my ankle, I allowed to myself, everything happens for a reason, so I guess moment was not the day for me to start running I 'll try again hereafter. So I did. That coming day I officially began my marathon training.

My excitement only
lasted for a many
blocks, as the physical
pain began to remind
me of what I believed
for so long I'm not a
runner. My hips pained.
My femur was sore. But
I was committed. I
completed my first
painful afar, but I
realized I demanded
help I demanded a plan.
I drove to the bookstore
and bought the perfect
book for me The Non-
Runner's Marathon
Trainer, by David
Whitsett. Now I had a
plan.

The first 10 days of
running were both
physically painful and
mentally grueling.
Every single day, I
fought a constant battle
in my head with the

voice of mediocrity, telling me it was okay to quit. But it was not. Do what's right, not what's easy, I reminded myself. I kept running. I was committed. Days 11-20 were only slightly lower painful. I still did not like running, but I did not really detest it presently. For the first time in my life, I was forming the habit of running every day. It was no longer this scary thing I only watched other people doing on the sidewalk while I was driving my auto. After nearly two weeks of diurnal handling, it was starting to feel normal for me to wake up every day, and just go for a run. I remained married. Days 21- 30 were nearly pleasurable. I had nearly

forgotten what it felt
like to detest handling. I
was doing it without
important study. I just
woke up, put on my
handling shoes(yes, I
had invested in a brace),
and logged my long
hauls each day. The
internal battle was gone,
replaced with reciting
positive declarations or
harkening to tone-
enhancement audios
while I ran. In just 30
days, I had overcome
my limiting belief that I
could not run. I was
getting what I would
have no way imagined
in a million times I was
getting a runner. Just 30
days after beginning the
habit of running
commodity that had
been so foreign and
unwelcome to me for
my entire life I had

completed 50 long hauls, climaxing in my first 6- afar run. I called Jon to celebrate. He was agitated for me, and always looking to help me raise my own norms, he presented me with a challenge. Jon knew me well enough to know that in the peak emotional state I was in, I would probably accept any challenge. "Hal, why do not you run an ultra-marathon? If you're going to run 26 long hauls, you might as well run 52. " Only Jon would suggest similar sense. "I'll suppose about it. " This time, when I told Jon I would suppose about it, I actually meant it. I was intrigued by the idea of pushing myself indeed further and running 52 successive long hauls. Perhaps Jon was right. If I was going to run 26, I might as well run 52. I mean, shoot, if I could go from running zero long hauls to being suitable to run 6 successive long hauls in just four weeks, and I still had six months until the Front Row Foundation's periodic Run for the Front charity run, why not set the bar a little advanced and go for 52? So I did. I was indeed ever suitable to move a friend and two of my stalwart coaching guests to do it with me! Six months latterly I had logged 475 long hauls, including three 20- afar runs, and had traveled across the country to meet with two of my favorite coaching guests James Hill and Favian Valencia, and long time friend, Alicia Anderer, so the four of us could essay to run 52   long hauls during the Atlantic City Marathon. Jon indeed flew out to show his support. There was just one logistical challenge though Atlantic   City was not set up for any "ultra" marathon runners. So, we extemporized. We met on the walk at 330 am. Our thing was to finish our first 26 long hauls before the sanctioned marathon began, also complete the second half with the regular marathon runners. The moment was surreal. The energy between the four of us was a mix of excitement, fear, adrenaline and unbelief. Were we really going to do this?! We might have been suitable to see our breath in the chill October air had the moonlight been lustrously. Nonetheless, our path was well enough lit, and so we began. One bottom in front of the other, one step at a time, we moved forward. We all agreed that was the key to our success that day keep moving forward. So long as we did not stop putting one bottom in front of the other, as long as we kept moving forward, we'd ultimately reach our destination. Six hours and five twinkles latterly, largely due to the collaborative support and responsibility of our group working together as one unit, we completed our first 26 long hauls. This was a defining moment for each of us. Not because of the twenty- six long hauls we had behind us, but because of the internal fiber it was going to take to get ourselves to run the twenty- six long hauls we had ahead of us. The excitement which percolated every fiber of our being just six hours before had been replaced with excruciating pain, fatigue, and internal prostration. Considering the physical and internal state we were in, we just did not know if we had it in us to duplicate what we had just done. But we did. Aggregate of 15 ½ hours from the time we started, James, Favian, Alicia, and I completed our 52- afar hunt together. One bottom in front of the other, and one- step at a time, we ran, jogged, walked, limped and literally crawled across the finish line. On the other side of that line was freedom the kind of freedom that can no way be taken down from you. It was freedom from our tone- assessed limitations. Although through our training we had grown to believe that running 52 successive long hauls was possible, none of us really believed in our heart of hearts that it was probable. As individualities, each of

us plodded with our
own fear and tone-
mistrustfulness. But the
moment we crossed that
finish line, we had given
ourselves the gift of
freedom from our fears,
our tone-
mistrustfulness, and our
tone- assessed
limitations. It was in
that moment I realized
that this is a gift of
freedom not reserved
for the chosen many,
but one that's available
to each and every one of
us the moment we make
the choice to take on
challenges that are out
of our comfort zone,
forcing us to grow, to
expand our capacity, to
be and do further than
we've been and done in
the history. This is true
freedom. The Miracle
Morning 30 Day Life

Transformation Challenge(in the coming chapter) will enable you to overcome your own tone-assessed limitations so you can be, do, and have everything you want in your life, faster than you ever allowed possible. The Miracle Morning is a life-changing diurnal habit, and while utmost people, who try it, love it from day one, getting yourself to follow through with it for 30 days so you can make it a lifelong habit will bear an unwavering commitment from you. On the other side of the coming 30 days is you getting the person you need to produce everything you've ever wanted for your life.

Seriously, what could be
more instigative than
that?

CHAPTER TEN

Forming habits that will transform accepting the challenge

Let's play devil's advocate for a moment. Can The Miracle Morning really transfigure your life in just 30 days? I mean, come on can anything really makes that significant of an impact on your life, that snappily? Well, flash back that it did for me, indeed when I was at my smallest point. It has for thousands of others. Ordinary people, just like you and me, getting extraordinary. In the last chapter you learned the simplest and most effective strategy for successfully enforcing and sustaining any new habit in 30 days. During The Miracle Morning 30 Day Life Transformation Challenge you'll identify the habits you believe will have the most significant impact on your life, your success, who you want to be and where you want to go. also, you 'll use the coming 30 days to form these habits, which will fully transfigure the direction of your life, your health, your wealth, your connections and any other aspect that you choose. By changing the direction of your life, you incontinently change your quality of life, and eventually, where you end up. When you commit to The Miracle Morning 30 Day Life Transformation Challenge, you'll be erecting a foundation for success in every area of your life, for the rest of your life. By waking up each morning and rehearsing The Miracle Morning, you'll begin each day with extraordinary situations of discipline(the pivotal capability to get yourself to follow through with your commitments), clarity(the power you 'll induce from fastening

on what's most
important), and
particular development (
maybe the single most
significant determining
factor in your success).
therefore, in the coming
30 days you 'll find
yourself snappily
getting the person you
need to be to produce
the extraordinary
situations of particular,
professional, and fiscal
success you truly ask .
You 'll also be
transubstantiating The
Miracle Morning from a
conception that you may
be agitated(and
conceivably a little
nervous) to " try " into a
lifelong habit, one that
will continue to develop
you into the person you
need to be to produce
the life you 've always
wanted. You'll begin to

fulfill your eventuality and see results in your life far beyond what you've ever endured before. In addition to developing successful habits, you'll also be developing the mindset you need to ameliorate your life both internally and externally. By rehearsing the Life S.A.V.E.R.S. each day, you'll be passing the physical, intellectual, emotional, and spiritual benefits of Silence, declarations, Visualization, Exercise, Reading, and Scribing. You'll incontinently feel less stressed-out, more centered, concentrated, happier and further agitated about your life. You 'll be generating further energy, clarity and provocation to move towards your loftiest pretensions and dreams(especially those you 've been putting off far too long). Flash back, your life situation will ameliorate after but only after you develop yourself into the person you need to be to ameliorate it. That's exactly what these coming 30 days of your life can be a new morning, and a new you. Still, or concerned about whether or not you If you're feeling hesitant. Will be suitable to follow through with this for 30 days, relax it's fully normal to feel that way. This is especially true if waking up in the morning is commodity you've set up challenging in the history. Flash back, we all suffer from RMS (Rearview Mirror Syndrome). So, it's not only anticipated that you would be a bit reluctant or nervous, but it's actually a sign that you 're ready to commit, else you would not be nervous. It's also important that you take confidence from the thousands of other people who have formerly gone from living on the wrong side of their implicit gap to fully transubstantiating their lives with The Miracle Morning. In fact, I'd like to take a moment to readdress and review a sprinkle of the Success Stories that were participated in the opening runners of this book. I really believe

the illustration of others can shine light on what's possible for us. I was so inspired by the metamorphosis that Melanie Deppen, an entrepreneur from Selinsgrove, PA participated with us "I'm on day 79 of The Miracle Morning, and since I began, I haven't missed a single day. Actually, this is the FIRST time in my life that I've ever set out to do commodity and have actually stuck with it for further than just a couple of days or weeks. I now look forward to waking up every day! It's inconceivable; The Miracle Morning has fully changed my life. "
I could not help but wish I had known about

The Miracle Morning
in council, or indeed
high academy, after
hearing the difference it
made for Michael
Reeves, a pupil from
Walnut Creek, CA "
When I first heard
about The Miracle
Morning, I allowed to
myself, ' this is so
crazy that it just might
work! ' I'm a council
pupil taking 19 units
and working full time,
so that left me with zero
time to work on my
pretensions. Before I
learned about The
Miracle Morning, I used
to wake up between 7-
9 am every day because
I had to get ready for
class but now I
constantly wake up at 5
am. I'm learning and
growing so much
through diurnal

particular development, and I'm LOVING The phenomenon Morning! ” Speaking of council scholars, Natanya Green now a yoga educator in Sacramento, CA began fulfilling her implicit with the help of The Miracle Morning while attending a California University “ After beginning The Miracle Morning in December, 2009, as a council pupil at UC Davis, I noticed profound changes incontinently. I snappily began to achieve long-asked   pretensions more fluently than I would have ever anticipated. I lost weight, set up a new love, attained my stylish grades ever, and indeed created multiple aqueducts of income all in lower than two months! Now, times latterly, The Miracle Morning is still an integral part of my diurnal life. " How could you not be impressed by the extraordinary position of commitment shown by Ray Ciafardini, a District Manager from Baltimore, MD "I 'm on my 83rd successive day of The Miracle Morning and just wish I had known about it sooner. It's amazing how important clarity I've throughout the day, now, thanks to The Miracle Morning. I'm suitable to concentrate on my work and all other tasks each day with so much further energy and enthusiasm. Thanks to The Miracle Morning, I'm passing a richer more abundant way of living in both my particular and my professional life. ” Eventually, I was blown down by the important story from Rob Leroy, an elderly Account Executive in Sacramento, CA “A many months ago, I decided to try The Miracle Morning. My life is changing so I cannot keep up! I ’m such a better person because of this and it’s contagious. My business was floundering, but after I started The Miracle Morning I was amazed at how, just by working on myself every day, I was suitable to turn it each around! ” Commit to and record your first Miracle Morning as soon as possible immaculately hereafter (yes, actually write it into your schedule) and decide where it'll take place. Flash back, it's recommended that you leave your bedroom and remove yourself from the   temptations of your bed altogether. My phenomenon Morning takes place every day on my living room settee while everyone differently in my house is still sound asleep. I've heard from people who do their Miracle Morning sitting outdoors in nature, similar as on their veranda or sundeck, or at a near demesne. Do yours where you feel most comfortable, but also where you won't be intruded Read the preface in your Miracle Morning 30 Day Life Transformation Challenge Fast launch tackle, also please follow the instructions, and complete the exercises. Like anything in life that's worthwhile, successfully completing The Miracle Morning 30- Day Life Transformation Challenge requires a bit of medication. It's important that you do the original exercises in your Fast launch tackle which should not take you further than 30- 60 twinkles) and keep in mind that your Miracle Morning will always start with the medication you do the day or night before to get yourself ready mentally, emotionally, and logistically for The Miracle Morning. This medication includes following the way in Chapter 5 the 5- Step Snooze- evidence Wake up Strategy. I n Chapter 3 the 95 Reality Check, we bandied the inarguable link between responsibility and success. All of us profit from the support that comes from embracing an advanced position of responsibility, so it's largely recommended but not needed that you get a suchlike- inclined responsibility mate to join you in The Miracle Morning 30 Day Life Transformation Challenge. Not only does having someone to hold us responsible increase the odds that we will follow through, but joining forces with someone differently is simply further fun! Consider that when you're agitated about commodity and committed to doing it on your own, there's a certain position of power in that excitement and in your individual commitment. Still, when you have someone differently in your life a friend, family member, or colleague and they're as agitated about it and committed to it as you are, it's much more important. Call, textbook, or dispatch one or further people moment, and invite them to join you for The Miracle Morning 30 Day Life Transformation Challenge. It'll bring them nothing, and you'll be teaming up with someone who's also committed to taking their life to the coming position, so the two of you can support, encourage, and hold each other responsible. IMPORTANT Don't stay until you have an Responsibility Partner on board to do your first Miracle Morning and start the 30- Day Life Transformation Challenge. Whether or not you've set up someone to embark on the trip with you, I recommend scheduling and doing your first Miracle Morning hereafter no matter what. Don't stay. You'll be indeed more able of inspiring someone differently to do The Miracle Morning with you if you've formerly endured a many days of it. Get started. Also, as soon as you can, invite a friend, family member, or colleague to visitwww.MiracleMorning.com to get their free phenomenon Morning "Crash Course." In lower than an hour, they'll be completely able of being your phenomenon Morning Responsibility Partner and presumably a little inspired. Are You Ready To Take Your Life To the Next Level? What's the coming position in your particular or professional life? Which areas need to be converted in order for you to reach that position? Give yourself the gift of investing just 30 days to make significant advancements in your life, one day at a time. No matter what your history has been, you can change your future, by changing the present.

CONCLUSION

Where you're a result of
who you were, but
where you end over
depends entirely on who
you choose to be from
this moment forward.
It's your time. Do not
put off creating and
passing the life
happiness, health,
wealth, success, and
love that you truly want
and earn for another
day. As my tutor Kevin
Bracy always prompted
"Do not stay to be
great." If you want your
life to ameliorate, you
have to ameliorate
yourself first. Get The
Miracle Morning 30
Day Life
Transformation Fast
launch tackle moment
atwww.TMMbook.com.
Also, with or without a
Responsibility Partner,
commit to your first

phenomenon Morning and beginning your 30-Day Life Transformation Challenge hereafter. You know, hereafter the day you begin your trip to creating the most extraordinary life you have ever imagined. If there's anything I can do to support you or add value to your   life in any way, please let me know.   Contact Me Anytimc I ’m always thankful to connect with like- inclined folks, and find it especially cool to hear from people who have read my books, seen my vids, or attended my speeches. So, if you have any questions or would just like to say hello, go towww.YoPalHal.com and click on the

"Contact" tab to shoot me a communication. I look forward to hearing from you, and exploring how I can add as important value to your life as I conceivably can. Let's Keep Helping Others May I ask you a quick favor? Still, if you feel like you're if this book has added value to your life. better off after reading it, and you see that The Miracle Morning can be a new morning for you to take any or every area of your life to the coming position, I 'm hoping you 'll do commodity for someone you love Give this book to them. Let them adopt your dupe. Ask them to read it. Or more yet, get them their own dupe, perhaps as a birthday or Christmas gift. Come to suppose of it what better book to give someone for Christmas than the only book that makes every morning feel like Christmas?! Or it could be for no special occasion at each, other than to say, "Hey, I love and appreciate you, and I want to help you live your stylish life. It was 2 o'clock in the morning. I could not sleep. Still renting a room from Matt, I was sitting at my cheap reproduction- pine office, crammed into my 12' x 12' living space. This smelled commodity had to change or perhaps I demanded to change. Gaping at my laptop and feeling frustrated with my life, I suddenly got inspired. I do not flash back exactly what urged it, but I opened up a new dispatch and started adding a veritably different group of people to the to field. Close musketeers, family, co-workers, former heads, and familiarity, the girl I was dating, and indeed believe it or not my ex-girlfriends. You name it; I was ready to make some radical changes in my life. I was ready for an amount vault in my implicit, and I felt the only way for me to get an accurate assessment of who I was, how I was showing up in my life, and where I demanded to ameliorate was to solicit honest feedback from the people who

knew me stylish. I
stopped when I got to
23 dispatch addresses,
because, well, I'm a
huge addict of Michael
Jordan and have a mild
preoccupation with the
number 23. I began to
compose an dispatch to
these people, who each
knew me in different
capacities and to
varying degrees,
explaining that I wanted
to grow tête-à-tête, to be
a better friend, son,
family, and coworker,
and that the only thing
to do was to get
feedback from people
who could see effects
about me that I could
not see about myself. I
asked if they would
please take a many
twinkles to reply, at
their foremost
convenience,

participating what they believed were the three biggest areas that I demanded to ameliorate. I asked that they be severely honest, and assured them that they would not hurt my passions. In fact, the only thing that would hurt my passions was for them to hold back, because doing so would only limit my growth. I'd be lying if I did not admit that this was the utmost whim-whams-racking dispatch I've ever composed. I nearly chickened out. I considered deleting it, and just going to bed. Thank God I did not. No, I took a deep breath, and I clicked shoot. Also, I went to bed, fell asleep, and awaited their responses.

Six hours latterly, I woke up. Stay, did I really shoot that dispatch at 2 o'clock in the morning, or was that just a dream? I logged into my dispatch. Nope, not a dream, I surely transferred it. And I formerly had two replies. One was from Mom, and the other was from. Brad Britton, a well- admired Region director at the 200 million bones Company I worked for. Oh boy, then goes I broke for an alternate and reminded myself that the purpose of this exercise was for me to grow and ameliorate, so no matter what anyone said in his or her dispatch, I was going to keep an open mind and not get offended. Easier

said than done. I
opened Mom's dispatch
first. Hey son, I got your
dispatch. (Really
mama? I had no idea
that you got it.) Well,
you know I suppose
you're perfect! But if I
must give you some
formative feedback, it's
that you should call
your mama more
frequently! I know
you're busy, but it
would be nice to hear
from you every
formerly in a while.
Anyway, I love you!
Come visit soon Love,
Mom. I opened up a
blank document on my
computer and named it
"Formative Feedback
and My New
Commitments. Call
Mom at least once a
week. Also I opened
the dispatch from my

Region director. Brad Britton. Brad is someone I respected and had learned a great deal from. Not to mention, he was one of the most positive people I knew. Although we only saw each other a many times throughout the time at conferences and on company passages, he knew me well, at least in a professional capacity. My confidante Hal! I love your dispatch. still, I'm only willing to give you the 3 pieces of " formative " feedback you have requested if you let me follow it up with 3 effects I like about you. Deal? Okay, then goes Brad progressed to enlighten me to a many of my professional and social "eyeless spots," all of which caught me by surprise. To be honest, my passions did get a bit hurt. I felt a little protective. That's not true. I 'm not really like that. He obviously does not know me as well as I allowed

also, it passed to me that it did not matter how accurate each of his examines were, because that was how I was showing up for him and presumably numerous others. It was important to me not just that I knew who I really was, but that I was living in alignment with my values, and harmonious in all of my connections. Dispatch responses continued to pour in over the coming many days. By the end of the week, 17 of the

23 donors had replied
with their thoughtful
and (substantially)
formative examine. I
had added a lot to my
"Formative Feedback
and My New
Commitments"
document since making
a note of my mama's
request for further
frequent contact. So,
what were the results?
Let's just say that I
gained more tone-
mindfulness and grew
further   in a week from
reading those responses
than I had grown in the
former 5 times
combined and
conceivably my entire
life. It was
inconceivable. It was
not easy to put myself in
such a vulnerable
position and look at all
of my excrescencies but

it was life- changing. It was career- advancing. It was relationship- perfecting. And it was all a result of mustering up enough courage to shoot what's presumably the most important dispatch that I've ever transferred The Dispatch That Will Change Your Life. Before I give you The Dispatch That Will Change Your Life below, word- for- word so you can copy, edit, and shoot it to your circle of influence I'd like to take a moment to partake some positive feedback with you from one of my guiding guests.

Problem Feedback avoidance. Utmost people do not enjoy

negative feedback, so they fully avoid asking for feedback. This prevents them from gaining inestimable data about their strengths and sins, therefore precluding them from staking on the former and significantly perfecting the ultimate. Result laboriously seeking and learning from the honest feedback of people who know you (in colorful capacities) is one of the most effective and fastest ways to gain a new perspective and accelerate your particular development and success.

Instructions Type the following textbook into an dispatch(feel free to edit and epitomize the dispatch so that it sounds like you.) shoot it to 5- 30 people(the further the better) who know you well enough to give you an honest assessment of your strengths and sins.